Weight Loss ASAP
Everything You Should Know!
(By Brian James)

Contents

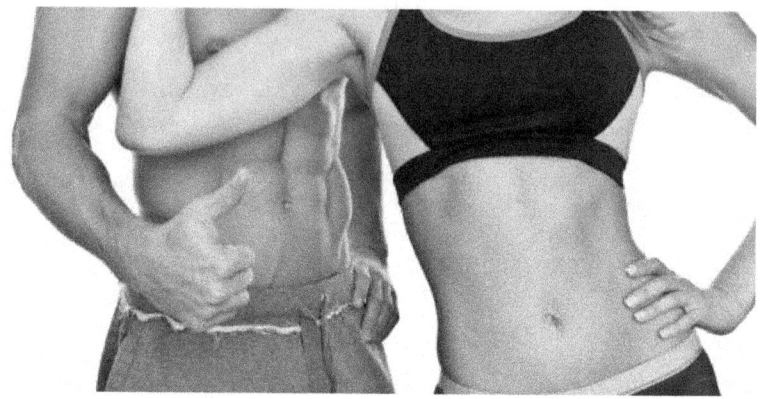

Introduction

Crash diets never result in long-term fat loss. In fact, they are more likely to be the source of long- term fat gain and are too hard to maintain. It will make your body to get low on energy and cause you to crave for high-fat and high-sugar foods. When you finally give up and eat those foods, the possibility is that you will consume more calories than you need, resulting in intense fat gain.

Over restriction of caloric intake and starving yourself will have the opposite effect on your body and will cause your body to go into starvation mode where anything you eat will store as fat, as your body will not know when will get food again. However, restricting calories to a healthy amount, and adding in exercise will help you to lose fat in long term.

The main thing to remember is that your body need at least 1200 calories a day to function and you burn them naturally throughout the day even without working out. In order to lose fat, stick to at least 1500 calories or maybe a little more if you start working out daily. Start your day with rich breakfast, have healthy snacks, healthy lunch and end it with little smaller healthy dinner, two hours before you go for goodnight sleep.

Always remember that fat loss is not an overnight process; as you didn't gain 10 lbs in a day. Therefore, you aren't going to lose 10 lbs. in a day either. Just keep with it and stay motivated, but by all means DO NOT starve yourself. It is really harmful for your body and will lead towards opposite effects. So instead stay motivated and follow healthy eating patterns. In general, any diet that requires eliminating 100% of signal type of food category isn't safe and once you are off of a fad diet the fat can return in no time.

It is always recommended by famous fitness expert to include snacks several times a day. It can support you with your fat-management goals because they provide essential energy, prevent overeating, and accelerate your metabolism.

Healthy snacks provide about 200 calories or less, and also contain a combination of nutrients and fibres. Always go for a snack that contains hunger-fighting protein, beneficial carbohydrates and heart-healthy unsaturated fat (found in nuts, seeds, fatty fish, oils, olives and avocadoes).

Moreover, avoid snacks that are nutrient-poor and provide calories from little to no beneficial nutrients like fibres, minerals and vitamins.

The word diet is not a very friendly word for your health. However, most people think that going on a specific diet is all they can do to make sure the fat loss. Cutting back on cookies and chips is a wonderful idea but dieting doesn't have to be about losing everything you love. Simply set yourself up with smaller portions at dinner and small dessert afterwards.

It is solely a doctor or dietician choice that can determine if you need to go on a true diet or not, but mostly they encourage a lifestyle and some eating pattern changes rather than depriving you of everything you love to eat.

Obesity has become a full fledge common disease these days. People tend to apply different remedies to loose fat instantly. Even latest technology is trying to incorporate several methods and techniques to enable people to get rid of flabby fat developed on their bodies. Some expensive methodologies like liposuction has also been introduced.

Only well-off people can avail this service due to its high cost. These are not the permanent ways of getting rid of fats. For the time being you might feel younger, slimmer and smarter but when the normal routine starts you again start to gain the unwanted fat.

Achieving best health through diet and exercise is not an overnight process. It requires systematic approach, well-defined goals and a planned health strategy.

The realization that you would start panting after a mild climb of three to four stairs is something to be worried about. The human body is the best possible form of a machine; but like other man made machines, this piece of intelligence and strength also requires constant maintenance and repair.

The main aspect of keeping your body healthy and active is the balanced diet and regular exercise.

Other variables like fat loss, aerobics, yoga etc. can guarantee a unique physique but the primary benefit lies in the diet you eat and the workout you perform to keep the heart running.

These days costs of medical services are soaring up to the sky. High medical bills can even leave you in debt and may lead you to inevitable stress and financial problems that can affect your body and mental health massively. Heading towards a healthy life through healthy means will enable you to live every day of your life at its best.

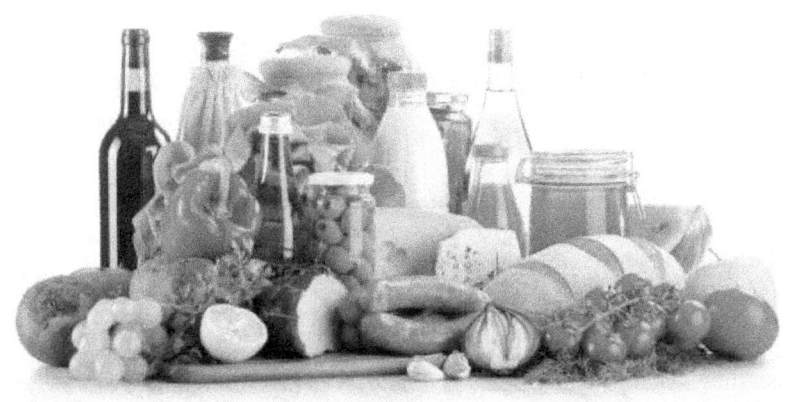

Chapter 1: Slimming Diet

Losing fat is not easy. It's like a slippery path where you have to walk very carefully. One wrong move and you slip down. As you learn what not to do while walking on a slippery path, you should also learn what not to include in your diet when you are trying to lose your fat. The lists of common foods you need to avoid are:

☐ Diet Soda
Many people think that having diet soda in their diet can help reduce fat but this is so not true. Diet soda contains many artificial sweeteners that play a role in increasing fat. People who want to lose fat should completely avoid it.

☐ Frozen food
Frozen meals might seem tempting when you are hungry. However, you need to know that those meals are loaded with salt in order to preserve them and as a result of that, your body demands more food and you need a large amount of water to dissolve that big amount of salt. It is, therefore, better to avoid them.

☐ White Rice
If you want to lose fat, you will have to say no to white rice. You can have brown rice instead. White rice has a low number of nutrients and that makes you hungry soon.

☐ White Bread

White bread makes your waistline grow bigger. It affects your blood sugar levels a great deal. It is better to avoid white bread if you are really serious about losing your fat.

☐ Ketchup

Ketchup contains high levels of sugar and salts. Ketchup and fries might seem to be a perfect-combo but ketchup and your waistline don't make a good combination. So, it's high time that you stop having ketchup often.

☐ Effect of Sugar

Sugar is good for health but when it comes to fat loss, you should probably quit consuming sugar. Sugar when consumed, converts into glucose and fructose. Glucose is very healthy for the body as our body produces it during metabolism. Fructose on the other hand, is not produced in the body and is not consumed by all cells of the body. Only the liver metabolizes and there it changes into fat.

☐ Effects of Raised Testosterone Levels On Fat Loss

Over fat people have low levels of testosterones. You can boost your testosterone levels naturally. Following is the list of few of the foods that can help you boost your
Testosterone levels:

- Citrus Fruits
- Eggs
- Red meat
- Avocado
- Beetroots
- Broccoli
- Pomegranate
- Watermelon
- Spinach
- Cabbage

Can Water Be Helpful In Losing Fats?
Researchers state that water does not magically help reduce fat. But, it indirectly is related to fat loss. Keeping yourself hydrated will help you prevent overeating because you feel full. Drinking cold water increases the metabolism rate. Therefore, drinking water can be somehow helpful in losing fat.

☐ **Small Meals Throughout The Day**
Losing fat doesn't mean that you should stop eating or you should eat when your stomach gets empty. You should have small healthy meals throughout the day.

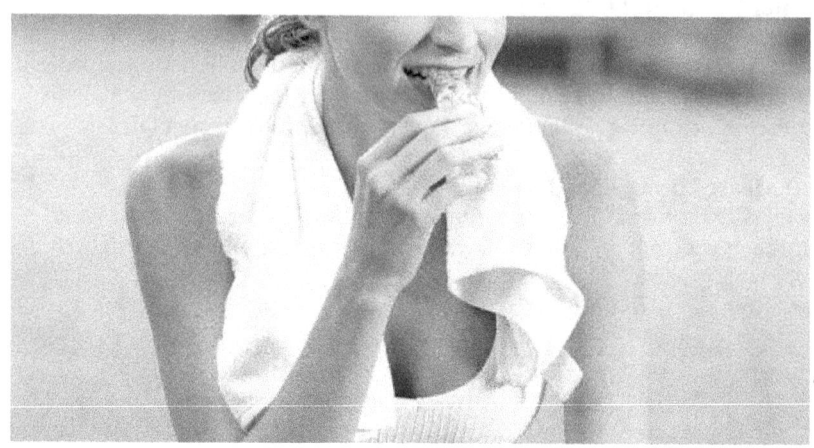

Chapter 2: Daily Habits of Healthy People

Fat loss is not as difficult as people say it is. It is definitely under your control, it's just that you have to make a proper plan to lose your fat. If you want to lose a hundred pounds in a few weeks then don't blame fat loss, it's your own mistake. Fat loss demands patience and dedication. You first have to change the lifestyle you are living. You will have to add things into your life that healthy people do. Here are a few things that you should do in order to lose fat.

☐ **Make a Calorie Chart**
You will have to make a calorie chart to check how many calories in a day, are you consuming. There are calorie calculators too that can better serve the purpose. You need to check out how many calories you need to consume in a day. You have to make sure that you don't starve. Once you are done with calculating the calories, the next thing you have to do is to distribute the calories, i.e. you have to divide the total number of calories in the meals you consume per day.

☐ Eat a balanced diet

Losing fat does not mean that you stop eating everything and starve to death. You need to know that if you are losing fat real quick, you will gain it real fast again. You have to include all carbohydrates, proteins and fats in your diet.

Sources
Proteins:
- Beef
- Chicken
- Eggs
- Fish

Low Carb Veggies:
- Zucchini
- Pumpkin
- Potatoes
- Corn
- Beets
- Peas
- Cabbage
- Carrot

Fats:
- Coconut oil
- Butter
- Olive oil

You should not be scared of consuming fat in your diet. Fish oil is a good thing to add in your nutrition plan. Do not starve yourself in order to lose fat.

☐ Eat slowly

You should quit eating fast. When we eat, a message is passed by the brain that we are full. This process takes a long while. If you eat fast, you will be full till your brain even processes the command. It is better that you eat slowly. This way you will not eat much. You will get full by having a little amount of food.

☐ Exercise

You definitely need to do exercise to burn calories but you should not do very strenuous exercises. You may burn a lot of calories while exercising but again if you eat a bowl of cereal, you will gain the double amount of calories again. You should only exercise for a little time. All you need to do is to put your focus on what and how much you eat. Start with 5 minutes a day and when your body gets used to it, increase the time. This is an effective way to lose fat. Just eat fewer calories and you are almost done.

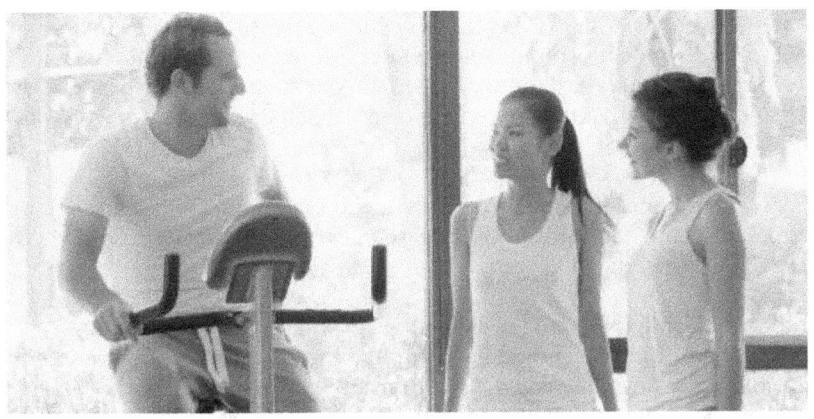

Chapter 3: Fat Loss vs. Weight Loss

You need to understand that weight loss and fat loss are not exactly same things. Weight loss is very easy to attain actually. All you need to do is to take in little amount of calories than what your body burns regularly.

If your body burns two thousand calories, and you just take in one thousand calories, you will probably feel that you are losing weight. The actual problem is that if the calories you are taking in do not have the sufficient amount of vital nutrients, the weight you are trying to lose may appear in the form of muscle tissue loss or maybe water weight. In the end you will observe changes but the result will be a more defined that what you thought it would be but you will see much smaller version of yours with a badly damaged metabolism.

Suppose that you follow a diet plan that generates a minor caloric shortfall. According to the plan, if you burn twenty five hundred calories each day, your body will consume twenty three hundred calories which means that you will face a shortfall of about two hundred calories every day. It doesn't sound healthy, right?

Now suppose that you are working under a good diet plan which consists of a good amount of carbohydrates, proteins and little amounts of good fats, and also once a week you much through a little more calories than the usual that will be about twenty six hundred calories so that you are able to prevent a metabolic slowdown. This sounds much better. Moreover, you craft an even larger caloric insufficiency all the way through your strenuous routines of body building and a cardiovascular plan which consists of a thirty minutes work out each day.

In this way, your bones and muscle tissues are conserved; in fact they get better and at the same time, fat loss and the release of extra water preservation are increased. This is clearly what we are trying to achieve.

It might look alluring to blame your metabolism when you put on large amount of weight. But you should keep in mind that as metabolism is a natural process; your body normally equalizes it to meet your particularized requirements. So, if you try your "starvation diets", your body balances by decelerating these corporal processes and preserves calories for body's survival. Only it happens in exceptional cases that you get unnecessary weight gain from a medical issue that results in slow down of metabolism rate, such as Cushing's syndrome or having an underactive thyroid gland.

Unhappily, weight gain is generally the outcome of having more calories than you burn. So, in order to lose weight you need to create an energy deficit by taking in smaller amount of calories, by raising the number of calories you metabolize by the help of bodily activities, or maybe both.

Restricting you calorie intake is almost a sure way to lose weight but you should remember to distinguish between weight loss and fat loss. This is something that applies anyone who is interested in bodybuilding or simply looking fit. You should work out more and more and have diet plan but you also need to be smart about it.

You do not have much power over the speed of your metabolism but what you can do is control the number of calories you burn b you physical activity. Simply put, the more active you are the more calories you will burn. Being more active is often mistaken for having a fast metabolism. You can be smart about your physical activity in the following ways.

□ Aerobic exercises are considered the most effective way to burn calories. These include walking, bicycling and swimming. You should at least try to inculcate 30 minutes of aerobic activity in your daily routine. If you are planning to lose weight or strengthen yourself then you probably need to increase this amount. If you cannot work out for a long period of time you can try another approach. This is to work out in separate sessions of 10-20 minutes throughout the day. This will promote activity for greater benefits.

☐ As you age you experience muscle loss. Any strength training such as weightlifting can help you counteract this loss. Another vital thing to consider is that muscle is excellent fat burners. So you should definitely consider adding muscle mass to reduce weight.

☐ Simple things like taking the stairs can or parking bit far at the store can help you reduce weight. Try to do anything that requires physical activity. You will only doing yourself a favor.

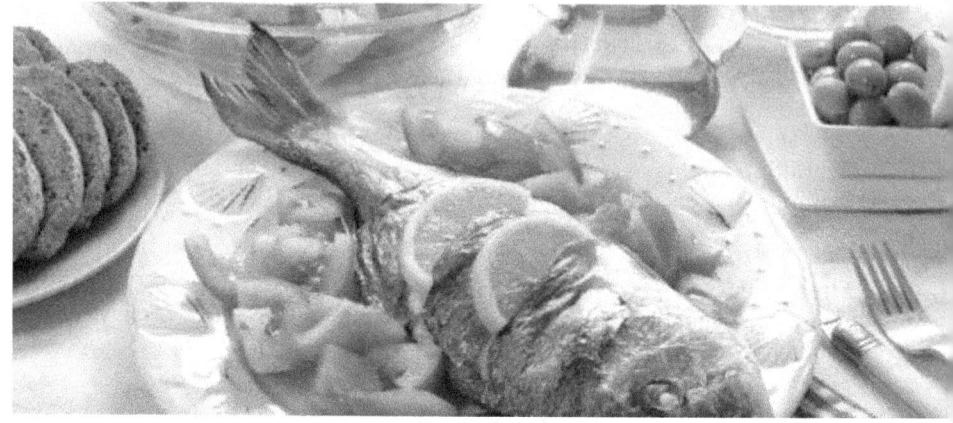

Chapter 4: Easiest Tips to Lose Fats

Naturally it is quite natural that everyone is trying to lose fat and also they want to lose it very quickly. Most of them try to take some diet pills, or switch to some fad diet, in order to lose fat. However the resulting fat loss is not long lasting. Many Studies have shown that people who lose fat gradually are more successful at keeping it off for long time. It is essential to change your lifestyle, in order to lose fat.

Therefore, if you do not have any habit to do exercise, then it is the most important recommendation to get start with it as soon as possible. You may become surprise by hearing that you can lose your fat in a natural way, without using any diet pills and fad diet. Natural fat loss is a very simple way for fat loss and it is not at all taking a diet pill or not about consuming fad diet. Mainly it is making gradual changes to your eating and lifestyle habits, due to which you lose fat and get health benefits.

1. Eat Vegetables
Five servings of vegetables a day steamed, raw or stir-fried are very important and consider it essential for your diet. A diet high in vegetables is linked with a reduced risk of developing cancers of the lung, breast, colon, cervix, esophagus, stomach, pancreas, bladder and ovary. Many of the most powerful phytonutrients are available in vegetables with the boldest colors such as broccoli, cabbage, tomatoes, carrot, grapes and leafy greens.

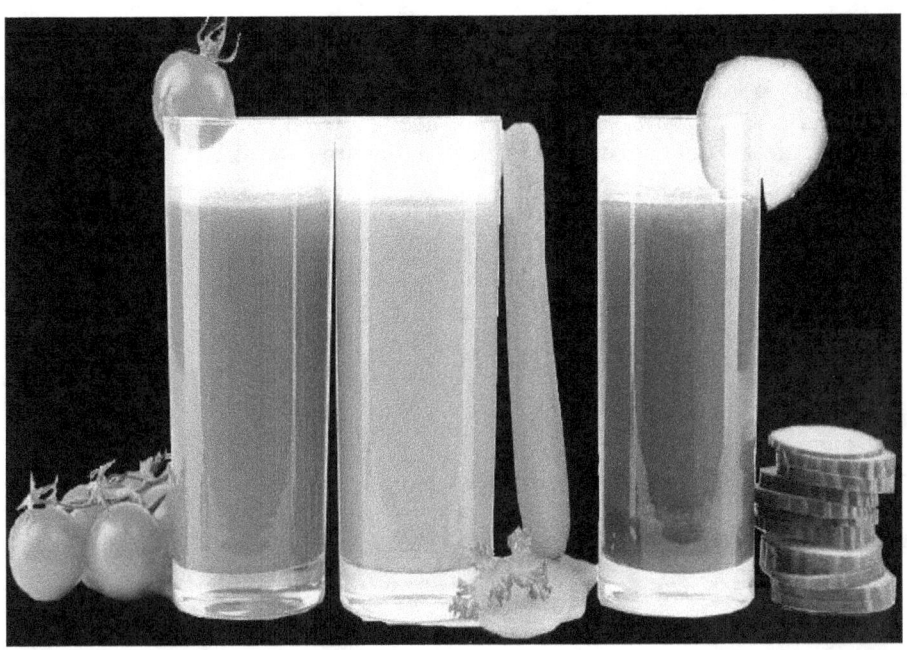

2. Exercise daily
This includes improving eyesight, normalizing blood pressure, improving lean muscle, lowering cholesterol and improving bone density. If you want to live well and live longer, you must exercise! Studies show that even 10 minutes of exercise makes a difference so do something! Crank the stereo and dance in your living room. Sign up for swing dancing or ballroom-dancing lessons. Walk to the park with your kids or a neighbor you'd like to catch up with. Jump rope or play hopscotch. Spin a hula hoop. Play water volleyball. Bike to work. Jump on a trampoline. Go for a hike.

3. Eat like a kid
If adding more fruits and vegetables sounds boring then look to "finger food" versions that preschool kids love such as celery and carrot sticks, cherry tomatoes, broccoli florets, berries, grapes and dried fruits. All are nourishing powerhouses full with antioxidants.

4. Use foods over supplements

Supplements are not a substitute for a good diet. Although many health experts recommend taking a multivitamin and mineral supplement that provides 100 to 200% of your recommended daily value, each and every supplement should be carefully evaluated for purity and safety.

Many supplements have been associated with toxicity, competition with other nutrients, reactions with medications, and even increased risk of diseases such as heart disease, cancer and diabetes.

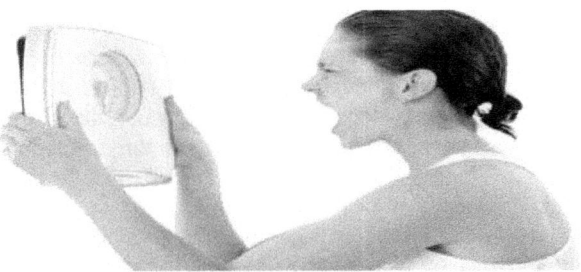

Chapter 5: 10 Reasons Why You Fail to Lose Fat

Achieving the best health and optimum fat through diet and exercise is not an overnight process. It requires systematic approach, well-defined goals and a planned health strategy. The realization that you would start panting after a mild climb of three to four stairs is something to be worried about. Human body is the best possible form of a machine; but like other man made machines, this piece of intelligence and strength also requires constant maintenance and repair.

The main aspect of keeping your body healthy and active is the balanced diet and regular exercise. Other variables like fat loss, aerobics, yoga etc. can guarantee a unique physique but the primary benefit lies in the diet you eat and the workout you perform to maintain the best body fat.

Fat loss is not an overnight process. It requires determination and patience along with momentarily patience. There is not just one reason that you are constantly failing in achieving a well-toned body. Incompetent in reducing your calories, not having a balanced diet, unable to cut down junk food and certain medical conditions can deteriorate your fat loss and fitness. Following are the reasons why you fail to lose fat:

1. Eating when you are not hungry – You are eating either you are bored, stressed out or emotionally upset. Most of the people want to fill up their mouths with food but doesn't want to fill up their bellies, which is totally illogical. Munching pointlessly for the sake of time pass will enable you to put on more fat. Some people eat chocolates when they are stressed out or undergoing emotional breakdown. What they don't realize is that besides the fact that chocolate is an anti-depressant, they are likely to gain fat more quickly in those days. People like to eat every time they sit in front of their TV screens.

2. Consuming more Calories than required – Keeping track of how many calories you averagely consume per day is very important. Set a threshold level against your fat and restrict yourself to consume calories above it. Maintaining a record should be an obligation to lose fat. Without proper check and balance you can also fall into over eating and fail to evaluate how many calories you consume daily.

3. Skipping breakfast – It is no myth that people who skip breakfast are likely to get more obese than those who start their day with a healthy breakfast. Breakfast enhances your metabolism, lowers your cholesterol level, vitalizes your energy, makes you more productive and improves your focus level. A healthy breakfast containing fibers and carbohydrates will help you prevent excessive hunger that can initiate overeating in lunch or dinner. The idea is very simple; if you starve yourself till lunch or dinner, you will definitely eat more and completely fail to lose fat.

4. Lack of Aerobic Exercise – One of the best ways to lose fat instantly is to perform aerobic exercises. 30 minutes of indulgence in aerobic exercises can burn handsome amount of calories. Eating three meals a day along with extra stuffing will give you many extra calories and the only way to burn them is through cardiovascular workouts such as running, cycling, trekking, skipping, jogging, swimming, and walking. Aerobics shall not only help you lose fat but intense workouts like stretching and strength training will give you more muscular strength and flexibility.

5. Lack of Muscle Building – The most effective method of burning fat and building muscle mass is strength training. Strength training affectively increases bone density, strengthens the heart, lowers pumping blood pressure, enhances blood flow activity, prevents degeneration of muscles, helps control blood sugar to an optimum level, improves cholesterol levels and tremendously improves your physical balance.

6. Excessive Perseverance Of Fluids – At times your body can start to retain water more than usual causing a serious condition known as edema. Edema is primarily caused by excessive salt in diet, severe medications, damaged or diseased liver or kidney, congestive heart failure, damaged lymphatic system, menstrual cycle, pregnancy and even hormonal imbalance.

7. Underactive Thyroid – Also known as Hypothyroidism, underactive thyroid plays a dramatic role against fat loss. People undergoing this medical condition will put on fat more quickly than those facing obesity. Underactive Thyroid is very common in both males and females aged from 40 to 50. Most common symptoms are hair fall, skin irritation, chronic fatigues, decline in immunity, sensitivity to cold, irregular periods, muscle and joint pains, regular cramps and muscle numbness.

8. Hormone Imbalance – This occurs when those hormones that actively participate in controlling fat are either outnumbered or are out of balance. Many doctors support the idea that balancing hormones level is the secret to fat loss, eliminating sleeping disorders, catalyst energy, stress life and active health. Certain factors revolve around hormonal imbalances, such as acne, hair problems, pregnancy, severe medications, malnutrition, infertility and menstrual problems.

9. Indigestion – There might be certain types of food that are unfit for your stomach and are unable to be digested by you. Even at time your stomach might show zero tolerance towards them, such as due to excess acidity in your stomach. Some foods can also cause fluid retention hindering your fat loss. Studies show that approximately 10% of adults are a victim of food intolerance.

10. Drugs, Supplements or Steroids – Certain medicines have noticeable side effects related very closely to fat gain or inability to lose fat. You need to identify which medicines, anti-depressants, oral contraceptives, supplements and steroids are restricting your fat loss.

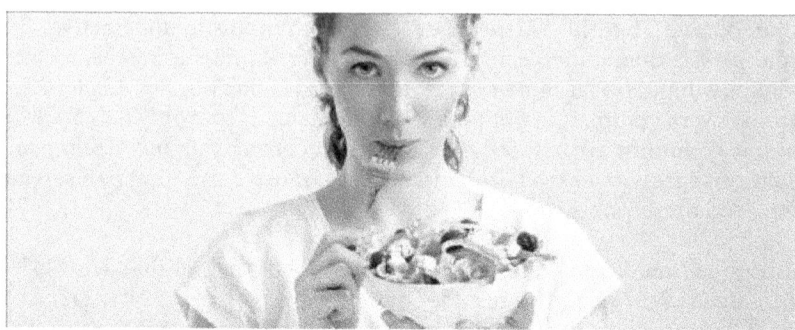

Chapter 6: The Diet Stress Factor

Generally, the new generation has stuffed their minds with the dieting and literally end up following a crash diet. Even if they are not fat or obese, they keep themselves on diet because of that peculiar "size zero" popularity.

Keeping yourself starved is not a good idea to get rid of the unwanted fats. Face is the first victim of diet. When you start dieting barely anything happens in the first phase, but the major difference you feel is your unattractive complexion and your weak face.

To run the race of losing fat you completely neglect or forget the other essential important things and trade off your looks on the first place. But avoid stressing yourself.

As it is so difficult to stick to the same diet, it makes you dull and bored. It is like doing something with immense pressure or utter compulsion. It is very difficult to maintain this but it is your will power that will carry you to the end.

At times people lose their mind to follow a diet plan. After the hard work of months and years, the not-expected result cause people intense disappoint and they lose their heart as well. No doubt, keeping oneself away from different types of tempting food requires a lot of sacrifice, patience and endurance.

Diet is not for the long run. You will get fed up of starving yourself. Who does not like to eat? Thinking of diet in your mind will make you stressed and anxious. Don't you know one of the things that make you gain instant weight is stress? The more stressed you are the more you will gain fat. Suppose you have an egg, pea, potato and walnut. Do you think you need one tool to cut them all? The answer is clearly no, because they all have different body types and structure. Likewise we all have different body types it is not possible to lose fat by doing same exercise and diet. People go on crazy diets and do not exercise at all. They just get themselves weak over a mal-nutritious diet plan.

It is not at all good for health. Our body needs specific amount of proteins and carbohydrates. Food gives you energy when and you utilize the food by working and exercising you can never get bad fats. Do you wonder why dieting is not helping you lose fat?

The common mistake is that you keep on starving yourself regardless of the fact that it gives you the unhappiness, you don't notice the main reason why you are gaining fat and it is definitely the anxiety, stress and depression caused by it. There is a strong connection of stress with the fat gain but few people realize this fact.

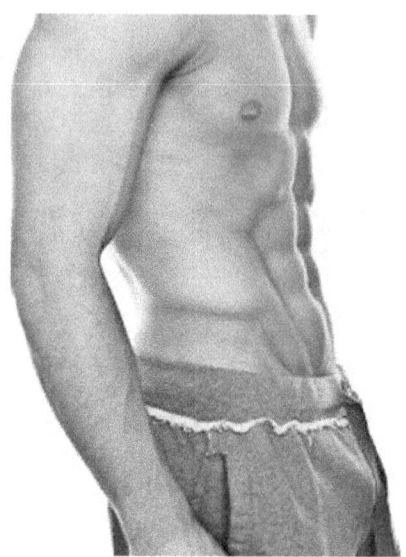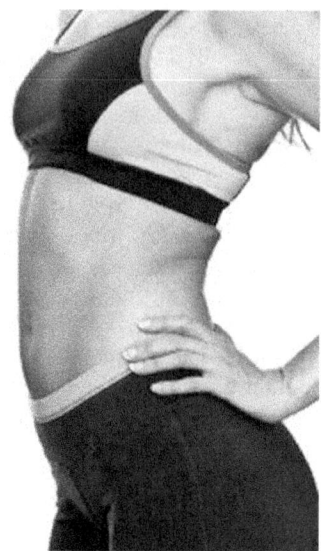

Chapter 7: Always Target Fat Loss

Fat reduction is complete process. It involves many steps. One of the most important steps is that you plan the whole process and do so intelligently and efficiently. You should set goals and targets in a specified manner so that you can stick to them better and cut that extra fat quickly and permanently.

You will see that most of the dieters mostly set goals and plans which involve demand. They try to make it a do or die situation. Their goals are loaded with words like "always", "never", "every" and "must". You should know that nobody is perfect.

When you imply demand like I swear I'll never have a doughnut or I'll never miss gym you are deliberately setting yourself up for failure because you are trying to be perfect. In most cases people who do this end up failing. This ends up in disappointment and demoralization.

Most people give up start again on their bad diet too. You should remember that to err is human. You should think practically. This will help you set realistic goals which are achievable. You will fell rewarded if you do so. There is another problem associated with setting goals. This is creating goals that are way too high. These goals are out of reach and not based on logical thinking. You here dieters saying that they will lose 50 pounds by the end of the month of they are going to walk ten miles a day.

These goals will overwhelm you because of the time they require and simply because they are gigantic. Another issue with this approach is that that you can only be successful when you complete the goal and the goal so impossibly large and far away that it mostly leaves people with despair.

This does not necessarily mean that your goals should not be challenging. They should be but huge goals are most likely to end up in failure. It is important to break down your huge goal into parts which you can accomplish easily and gradually. This will build you morale and help you feel rewarded too.

Setting goals and organizing yourself is a perfect way to get started. They can be used to use your time better and spend energy on required areas.

☐ Your goals should be short term and specific. They should mostly comprise of what you are going to do tomorrow or next week. They should specify exactly what you plan to do so can have clarity.

☐ The goals you set should be traceable. You can track them by keeping a dairy or journal. This helps you see your progress and motivates you too.

☐ Your goals should exhibit positivity. This will further enhance your morale. They should be "I will" rather than "I won't". Negative goals will leave you with a sense of depravity.

☐ Try not to lose fat for others. Do it for yourself so that you can do it better.

☐ Appreciating the journey is important. You should reward yourself in some way after every small victory.

☐ Your goals should be realistic so that you can have long-term success. You can live with these goals and make them a part of your life.

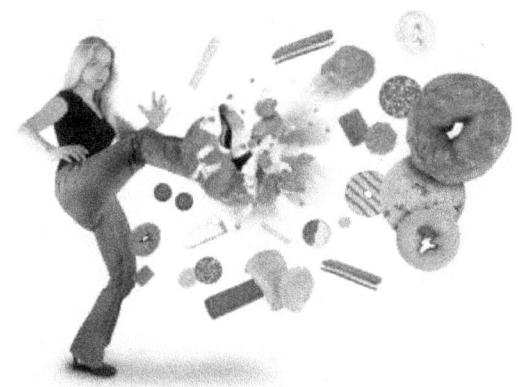

Chapter 8: Myths about Fat Loss

The human body is built to survive. It slowly adapts in order to persist in tough conditions. It has evolved in to a fat piling machine. Our bodies store the food that is not immediately used for energy as fat. This fat is converted back in to energy for our brain and muscles when our food intake is not enough. For the ancient human this was a very helpful ability.

But in today's time when food is abundant this is a serious issue for us.
The global increase in obesity and high fat is due to a number of factors, but whatever the factors maybe maintaining a healthy fat is vital. In order to lose fat our body must use more calories than we eat or drink.

Fat loss has been brought up as a serious issue worldwide and many people are now considering this as an actual problem. More and more people are committed to fat loss.

We will be looking at the top myths associated with fat loss.

☐ **Starving can result in fat loss**
Starving yourself is probably the worst way to lose fat. These crash diets have no results in the long run. Starving yourself can even lead to fat gain. The biggest issue with this type of diet is that you cannot maintain it. As you starve

yourself the energy level decreases. This causes you to yearn for high-fat and high-sugar foods and when you finally give in to your hunger you will probably eat more food than you really need. So this approach can end fat gain.

☐ A vigorous exercise is the only way to lose fat
Many people are still of the opinion that strenuous exercise is the only way to lose fat. In order to successfully control your fat, changes in your physical activity must be small and gradual. Normally an adult between 19 and 64 at least need 150 minute of physical activity, every week. Over fat individuals probably need more than this. Using more calories than you are eating can cause you to lose fat. Exercise burns more calories and eating less decreases the intake. You should have sound combination of the two to lose fat.

☐ Slimming pills have long-term effects
Slimming pills are not a way to lose fat affectively. They should only be used when prescribed by a doctor. Other than that these pills can also have wide array of side effects. Long-term fat loss cannot be achieved by pills.

☐ Putting a halt to snacking can help you lose fat
People who have an active lifestyle need a snack in-between meals to maintain their energy level. Snacking is not a problem when you are losing fat. The thing that matters is the type on snack. You should try and consume fruits and vegetables rather than chocolates or crisps which have high sugar and saturated fat.

☐ You can lose fat by drinking water
Water cannot help you lose fat. Water is necessary for your optimal health. It also keeps you hydrated. When you are hydrated you are less likely to snack. People often mistake being thirsty for being hungry so if you are not hydrated you may eat more. You need at least 1.2 liters of water daily. Water keeps you hydrated and does not help you lose fat.

☐ You can lose fat by skipping meals
If you are trying to lose fat skipping meals is not a good idea. Losing fat means that you have to reduce the intake of calories or increase the burning of calories. When you skip meals you are likely to feel tired and you will suffer from malnutrition. High-fat and high-sugar snacking can result in such a situation which will only result in fat gain.

☐ Carbs are not helpful for dieters

Carbohydrates are a great source of energy. All Carbs are not equal. Low-carb diets are vital. You just need to limit the amount of processed carbs such as white bread or croissants. You can enjoy beans and whole grains such as brown rice and whole-wheat bread. Fruits and vegetables are rich in nutrients and fiber and low in calories so they help reduce risk of obesity and heart disease. Carbs also help you burn body fat.

☐ Frozen fruits and vegetables are not as nutritious as fresh ones

This is another myth associated with dieting. Fruits and vegetables picked at the peak of ripeness are full of more vitamins and minerals. The amount of nutrients drops as they are shipped and stored. Frozen products are flash frozen so they are almost as full of nutrients as fresh ones. Frozen products without added sugar, syrup, sauce or cheese have less calories.

☐ Not having breakfast will help you lose fat

This is a common practice among novice dieters. They assume that by not having breakfast will help them control their fat. According to a recent British study which consisted of 6,764 people who skipped breakfast gained twice as much fat over the course of four years as breakfast eaters. Speaking of skipping breakfast it must also be mentioned that skipping any meal will cause you to gain fat.

☐ Your fat and metabolism is determined by your genes

This is also a big myth associated with fat issues. Most obese people argue that their fat is a cause of their heritage. This is false concept. Only 25 percent of your body fat is determined by your genes. You can lower your fat by combining low-calorie diet and exercise. Metabolism can also be increased by performing strength and resistance exercises.

☐ The best time for exercise is early morning

People often argue that exercise done in the morning is much more useful. This is a false assumption. You will benefit the same amount and burn the same number of calories whenever you work out. The important thing to remember is to keep doing it regularly.

Depending whether you have free time in the evening or morning you can work out whenever you want. The key thing is that you do.

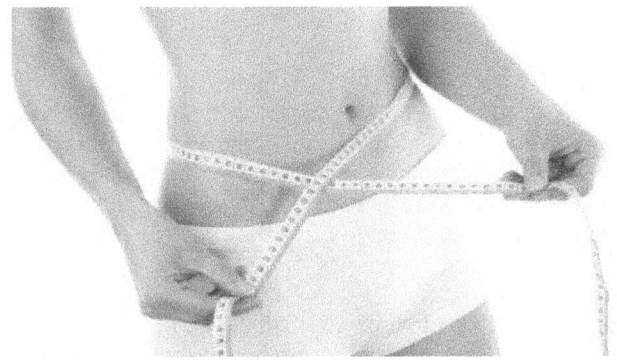

Chapter 9: Fasten Up Your Motivation

Belts to Lose Fats

So if you have set your fat goal and have planned out your exercise routine by becoming a member at your local gym, then now is the time to maintain that level of enthusiasm to reach your fat loss goals and objectives. But the question at hand is that your fat loss motivation starting to wane?

Don't fear anything at all under any circumstances. Remember motivation and persistence is the key to nail every fat loss goal. No matter how daunting fat losing tasks seems to be but few simple techniques can keep you motivated for the long haul and allow you to have fun in the process, as Jillian Michaels once said "Until you puke, faint or die, keep going".

Many of us remain unable to follow long lasting diet and exercise plan, so we have gathered best inspirational tips from world's top dieticians, doctors, life coaches and fitness experts for staying motivated to lose fat.

☐ Maintaining Your Diet
Never fall in the trap of crash diets, have often claimed to be carb-free or all-protein recipes they are unnatural and bound to be short-lived. Trust us you will be more motivated with the diet that makes you feel and look good then diet that involves severe calorie limitations. Are you craving for desert while following a specific diet plan? Add a little portion of it in your daily diet. If you

can't have it at all, you'll want it even more therefore instead of eliminating it.

☐ Avoid Emotional Eating

When we are happy, we eat. When we are depressed, we eat. When we have nothing else to do we eat and worst of all is that these diet habits will take you nowhere near your fat loss goal. It is compulsory to identify and analyze your eating patterns and start by keeping your hands busy, by knitting, reading, or doing a word puzzle; hence, it will restrain you from grabbing any junk food.

☐ Keep a Food Journal

Write down everything you eat to keep a record of what you're eating and notice your bad eating habits. Also get a food journaling partner if possible because eating 4 cookies is a lot more embarrassing when you have to tell someone else about your dirty deed.

☐ Sticking to Your Workout Plan

It is harder to skip gym or yoga session, if you know there is someone waiting for you to meet them at the fitness studio or at the start of a jogging route. Therefore, friends and family can be excellent motivators and offer support along the way and can even become participants alongside you, when you continue toward fat loss goal.

Remember that not every form of fitness geared towards fat loss is limited to your daily workout. Preserving or pursuing a healthy body fat includes making physical activity by swapping few patterns in your daily activities for example in order to reach fat goal faster, choose to take the stairs over the elevator.

Moreover, these little changes will not only benefit your waistline but also moving frequently can alleviate feelings of sluggishness and motivate you to continue moving throughout the day. To excite a drab workout, a new iPod, new music and a new water bottle will do the trick.

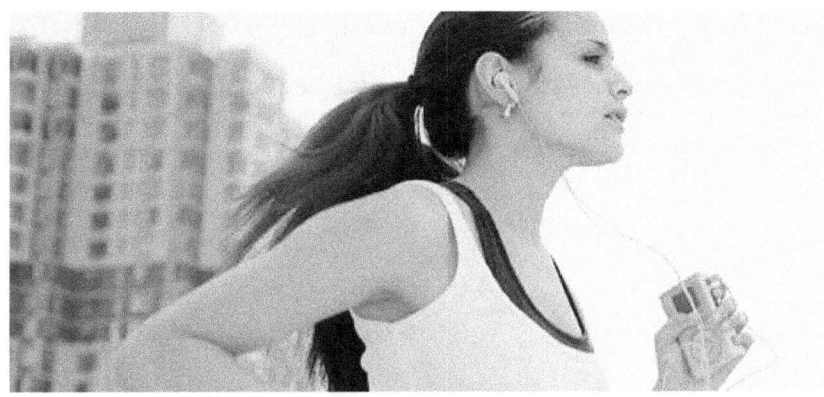

Chapter 10: The Mighty Metabolism

Do you know when you do not eat timely and properly a hormone known as 'ghrelin' is secreted in the stomach to ensure that we eat. The release of ghrelin is an involuntary action and is under no one's control.

So you should take your meals 4-5 times a day. It keeps your metabolism active and fast. Metabolism is the process by which anything you eat converts into energy. A slow metabolism is the cause of excess fat gain. When you are on diet and are not eating properly, your body will require nutrients, proteins and carbohydrates. When it does not get the proper amount of nutrients it slows down the process of metabolism and stores food in the form of fats.

You can increase your body metabolism through adjusting your eating habits by in taking small and frequent meals. When the time period between your meals extend it decreases your metabolism. Keep your body hydrated. Drink at least 3 to 4 Liters of water daily. It will primarily help in the detoxification by keep eliminating the waste toxics from the body.

Different physical activities like cycling, running, hiking, trekking and other aerobic exercises will impressively boost up your metabolism. Increased metabolism in turn will encourage fat loss quickly.

Remember, while performing any special physical activity or taking any medicine always consult your physician, nutritionist or health care professional. At times, people tend to hurt themselves with exerting a lot of stress on body mass and muscles during exercising.

Always maintain a steady balance while performing any sort of physical workout. Exercise is a good thing but excess of anything can prove to be very harmful for the health.

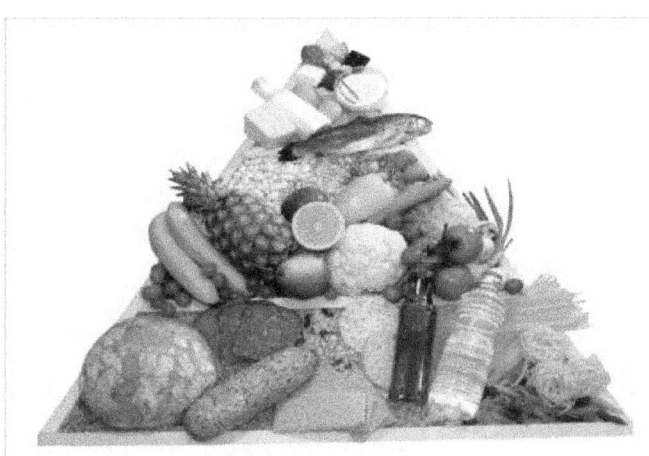

Chapter 11: The Ultimate Balanced Diet

Combination of a balance diet with good exercise will prevent your body from fatigue or unnecessary exhaustion, enabling you to build an overall stable stamina. Your body needs proper balanced diet consisting of all sorts of foods like fruits, vegetables, eggs, milk, meat, and bran.

Several research studies have shown that there are three types of human bodies. The first type is the one who eat too much but they do not gain fat. They are naturally skinny and are known as Ectomorphs.

The second is those with the thick body type. Despite of their crash diet and regular exercise, they do not lose fat and are known as Endomorphs. The third type is called Mesomorph. They are in between Ectomorph and Endomorph. They are the ones with perfect body and get in to the tune they want. Most common examples of this type are the athletes, models, celebrities, fitness experts and bodybuilders.

After knowing the fact that you belong to three different body types. So do you still think all of you can lose fat and gain perfect body with the same diet? Just know the fact and keep going slowly; believing that no good thing comes instantly. If it is an instant affect then it might be not reliable or suitable for your body type. Increase your metabolism to kick off the unwanted fats. With the hard work slowly and steady you will see the tremendous changes taking place.

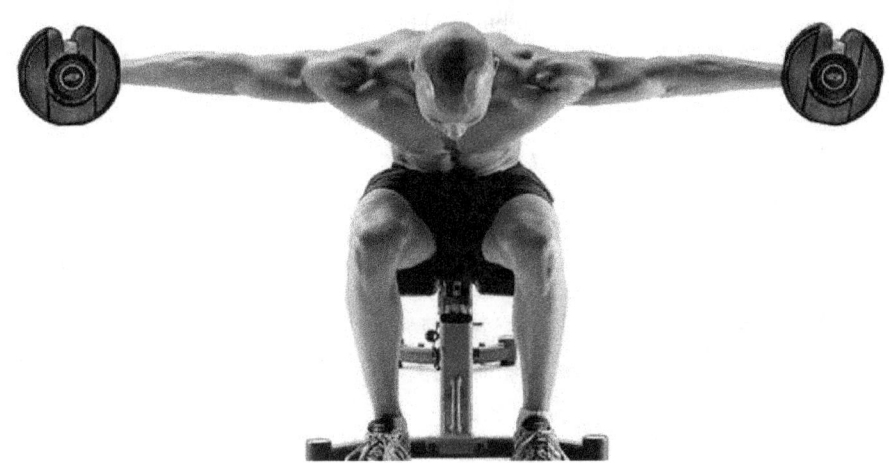

Chapter 12: Working Out For A Slim & Sleek Body

Some recent hype about how exercise won't make you slim is surely a misguidance to all the fat watchers out there. If you are new to this entire fat reduction world you get one thing down. There is no way that you can reduce fat without working out. Exercise is not only crucial to fat reduction it also forms a part of a healthy and balanced lifestyle.

To reduce fat a healthy diet must also be accompanied by work out plan and good amount of physical activity. It is proven fact that you need to work out to lose fat. Countless studies and all experts agree with the fact that working out works if you are trying to reduce your fat. Exercise is suing shot way to keep you fit, slim and happy.

Most people wanting to reduce fat have surely a big round belly. To make things simple, the only way to zap that belly fat is to work out. High intensity or even regular moderate intensity aerobic exercises will have the most effect on your abs. This is the fat that poses a potential risk to diabetes and heart diseases. Cortisol is a hormone which is linked to b fat, working out acts as a moderator in order to lower the levels of this hormone to help you reduce your belly fat. So not only do you tone your body you also protect your heart against many diseases.

If simply put losing fat is all about burning more calories than you are consuming. Exercise helps you burn all that stored fat in your body to help you ease up on your fat. Excess fat can only be burned by physical activity of the vigorous sort. You continue to burn calories hours after you have stopped working out. Fats stored in your body can be harmful and working out removes it.

Another reason why it is crucial to work out is that it helps you maintain your fat after you have lowered it. Exercise is even prescribed to people who undergo fat reduction surgeries to help them keep that figure. An hour of exercise of daily helps you keep off the fat you have lost. So working out is not only to help you reduce fat it also ensures that you keep that fat steady so you should keep it in mind that if you want to have that ideal figure you really need to work out.

Another benefit of working out is that is boosts up your metabolism. When you eat less you are sure to lose muscle. This means that you will also burn fewer calories. Exercise helps you build muscles. These muscles when combined with a high metabolism will help you torch a lot of calories.

Working out not necessarily will decrease your fat. It can help you build muscles. Another advantage of working out is that it even helps you build a positive attitude. Exercise helps you regulate your mood so when you are upset or stressed you should work out rather than eating.

It is a general fact that positive activities will further cultivate healthy habits. When you are working out to healthier lifestyle you will automatically be directed to further you struggles in order to better yourself.

Compound exercises area much more affective for fat reduction. These are the exercises which involves more than one major muscle at a time. Exercises which involves pushing, pulling, squatting or deadlifting it is a compound exercise. Compound exercises engage more muscles which in turn gives you better results.

Another thing you can do to lose fat quickly is sprint instead of jog. A 40-45 minute jog has about the same effect as 3 or 4 sprinting sessions which usually take 10-20 minutes.

Sprinting is considered a high intensity workout. It helps you achieve a lot more in much lesser time. So you should consider sprinting instead of long jogs to lose more fat in less time.

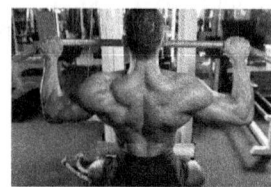

Chapter 13: Muscle Building

You hear it all the time. Eat right and work out if you want to lose fat and start living healthy. What we are going to discuss is really important. You might spend a lot of time jogging or on light work outs. This is helpful but not helpful enough.

If you want to burn a lot of calories and fast then you really need to build lean muscle. It is fact that fat training helps you burn much more calories. Building muscles must be a major priority in your workout routine.

Cardiovascular exercises do help you burn fat but only while they are being performed. But when you have muscles your fat burns to sustain the body. Having muscles help you burn fat even in the most mundane task like walking. Muscle burns more calories because it requires more energy than fat. Cardio only burn fat when you are working out but muscles burn calories around the clock.

Vitamin D is nutrient in the body which is rapidly depleted. Working out in the open can be great way to build your muscles and help you stock up on that lost vitamin D. Vitamin D comes from sunshine so you should consider exercising in the open to help produce vitamin D.

You can head up to your local park and do pull ups of pushups. Another great way to spend time in the sun and work out is to try out organized activities like rock climbing or marathons. They can provide you with a workout and entertainment at the same time.

The possibilities and choices of outdoor activities are limitless. You just need to do something that adds resistance to your muscles. The important thing is that you get up and find it in yourself to actually do stuff which puts strain on your body so you can start cutting that excess fat.

It is not mandatory to work out only outside. You can exercise at your home too. The thing is to be consistent. Muscle building will not only help you lose fat but it will also strengthen you and help you better your posture. It straightens out your back too.

Working out has endless benefits. The primary energy consumer in our bodies is the muscles. Your body is like a big fire. Fat burns slowly. Compared to that muscle require more energy and so it consumes much more calories. Adding more muscles to your body means that you will lose much more energy and less fat will be stored in your body.

Muscle building is better than cardio exercise as it consumes more calories. Muscles increase your metabolism, when you have boosted metabolism your muscles burn calorie every time you make a movement.

Muscles are in constant need of calories even when you are doing very little physical activity. Just to sustain itself a pound of muscles needs about 50 to 150 calories a day. In comparison to this a pound of fat requires 1 to 3 calories. As your muscles increase your metabolic rate increases and so does your daily calorie burn.

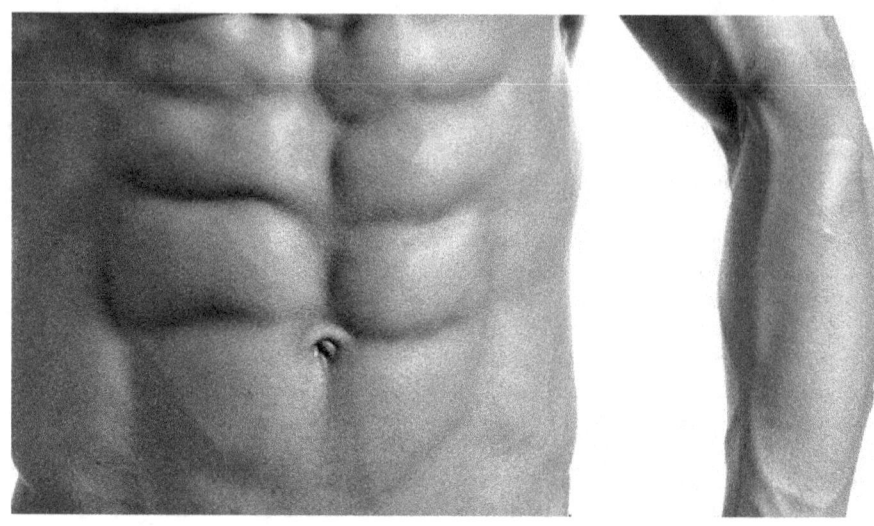

Chapter 14: Six Pack

Whenever you think of muscle building the first that comes to anyone's mind are the six packs. Apart from the attractiveness of the six packs they also provide you with a wide range of medical benefits.

The medical benefits of six packs are majorly underrated, when you have strong abdominal muscles, meaning that you have a six pack you far less likely to suffer from back injury. Back problems are pretty common these days. You hear a lot of people complaining about lower back pain. This pain is mostly associated with weal abdominal muscles and a large amount of belly fat. Having a six packs and strengthened abs can significantly reduce the risk of back aches and other injuries which are due to belly fat and disproportionate fat distribution.

Another common issue related to weak abs is a hernia. This is due to the weak abdominal wall. Fascia is the connecting muscle tissue which overlays the stomach. Hernia is when the fascia is breached by organs or other fatty tissues. When the wall is breached the muscle tears and parts of intestines are pushed outwards. This creates a bulge which is both painful and unbearable. A hernia can only be surgically corrected. After the surgery you can permanently kiss your dream of six pack goodbye because you can't lift any heavy objects without the risk of serious injury. Joint pressure is also a serious issue. Having a strong abdomen and strong muscular physique is an excellent way to decrease pressure on the joints to stabilize the body. Joint pressure can become a serious issue with growing age. So having six packs can help you divert an incoming problem.

You can also enjoy the benefits of heightened stamina with six packs. You have to stay fit and work out on regular basis to have a six pack. This gives you the ability to sustain physical exertion for a longer period of time without getting tired. They also get to keep peak physical performance. This can may benefits as you can easily maintain a healthier and active lifestyle.

You also enjoy a better posture with six packs. A muscular abdominal coupled with a smaller waistline can help you stand up straighter rather than hunching over. Upper and lower back pains and spinal complications are a common result of bad posture.

You also look much better standing and walking. Better posture can also make you look taller. So there you have it, having six pack not only looks good but it also has numerous medical benefits.

From preventing hernias to improving your posture, six abs can have big impact on your health. Working on your abs will also improve your metabolic rate which in turn will burn more calories so you can cut fat. So if you are working out to lose fat you are well on your way to very healthy life. Clothes also look better with six packs.

Only having six pack has so much advantages then you can imagine what a toned body would be like.

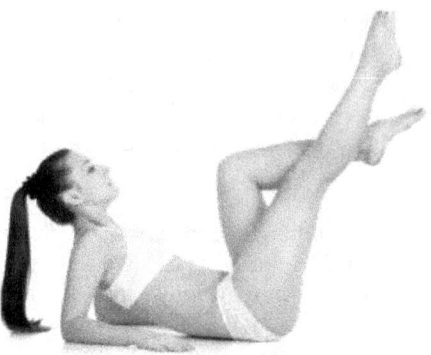

Chapter 15: Fat Loss Surgery For Ultimate Slimming

Another practice common now a days is fat loss surgery. This is an extreme measure and should only be considered a last resort. This is mostly prescribed to patients with extreme cases of obesity. Like all surgical procedures this surgery also comes with risks. This type of surgery is termed as bariatric surgery. Mostly, it is of two types:

First type is gastric bypass surgery. Many complications have been associated with gastric bypass. On such complication is "dumping syndrome". The patient may suffer from nausea, abdominal cramping, and diarrhea after eating sugar. It may also include weakness or faintness. Other complications include narrowing or ulcer formation or leak at the stomach to intestine connection. If this occurs reoperation is required. Open bariatric surgery can also cause incisional hernia.

Blood clots in the leg are also found in some patients. They can eventually migrate up to lungs causing complications. These are surgical complications. The patient may also suffer from long term issues. This is due to the malabsorption if the patient does not take supplemental nutrients. These deficiencies include.

☐ Vitamin deficiencies (A, B-12, D, E, and K). Deficiencies of vitamin B-12, folate, and iron can cause anemia.

☐ Mineral deficiencies (calcium, iron, and folic acid) - Calcium deficiency is a concern because it may lead to osteoporosis and other bone disorders.
The second type of fat loss surgery is gastric band. It can also have some serious affects.

Patients suffering from gastro esophageal reflux disease (GERD) or who are sweat eaters cannot have a lap-band system type of operation. There is also a small possibility of port leak or infection, slippage, erosion or migration of the band altogether. Reoperation is required in these cases. Mostly gastric band cases are converted to gastric bypass this may also reflect the surgeon's learning curve.

Some patients may also regain fat after their surgeries. This can occur due to number of reasons. Patients do not follow the diet prescribed to them after the surgery. Some patients neglect the importance of postoperative exercise which results in their fat gain.

Stretching of the pouch is also associated with fat gain. Communication issues between the pouch and the stomach may also occur which lead to fat gain. The band may induce issues to revert the fat loss too.

One more thing to consider is the actual amount of the surgery. It is much more expensive than other treatments for obesity. So you should rely on surgery only as the last resort.

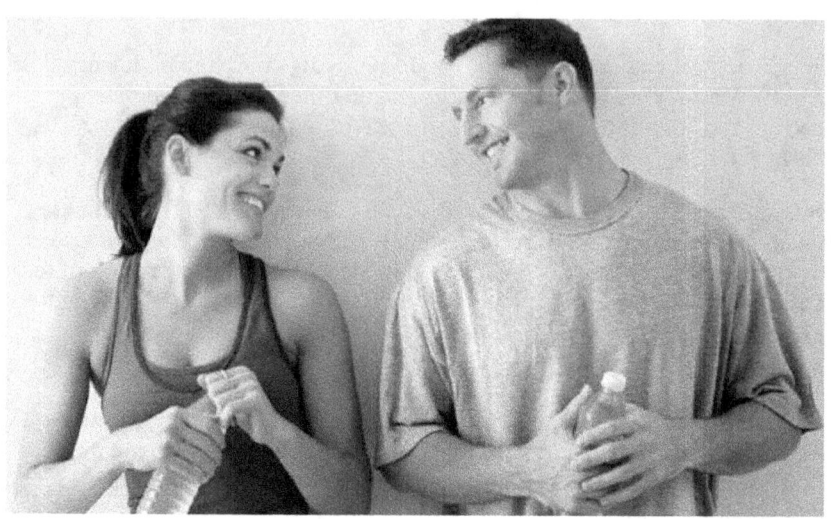

Chapter 16: Get Slim with Friends

I have always gotten the impression that if you want to lose your fat all over; you need to make friends who can keep a check on what you are doing. Make fitness partners. A study states that working with someone on a job increases the performance in the long run.

When you have a friend with you, who has the same goal as you have, you will enjoy losing fat and you will do more and more in order to compete with your friends.

Your partner and you can set different goals. When you achieve your goal, you can celebrate it. If someone fails to achieve it, he will have to give a treat as a punishment to the other one. Many people say that having a fitness partner has a great impact on your failure or success in any fitness plan.

Kenneth Schwarz says, "In the realm of dieting, there is evidence that social support is a positive factor influencing fat loss." You can count on your diet buddy because you share a common goal. If you work with someone who motivates you, you will squeeze more and more out of you.

There is no need to worry if you do not find a fitness buddy. There are many smart phone apps that too can serve the purpose. Almost all the smart phone apps have fat loss apps that can be very helpful. You can set a particular time and your smart phone will remind you about the routine.

You can use the apps to calculate how many miles you have walked or for how long did you do the exercise. This way you will have a check on what you are doing.

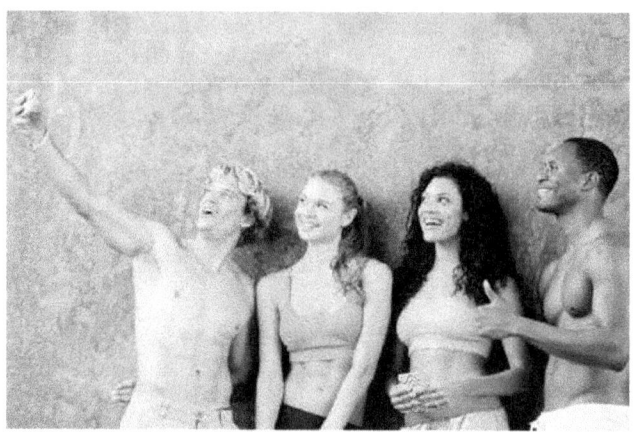

Chapter 17: The Social Circle Slimming

When trying to cope up with fat gain or obesity some people lack the ability to appreciate what it means to have support and motivation along the way. Human beings are social animals. We live with people and we absorb their recommendations, feelings and opinions.

For some people the whole idea of reducing their fat is to be accepted by those around them. This maybe a false ideology but for some it is a source of continuous motivation.

Support from your social circle can have a tremendous effect on your fat reducing regime. You might be a little hesitant to tell your family and friends about how you plan to take on healthier form of life. This is particularly hard when you have tried to reduce your fat in the past and you have failed to do so. Don't be.

Think of it this way. They are the ones who care for you and want the best for you. When they know about your goal and the factors affecting your fat reduction they will support you in your struggle.

You don't have to stay motivated on your own. They will also take measures to help ensure that this process is easy and fun for you. Your friends might join your fitness sessions. Your family can help by preparing meals for you that are healthier. They can give you motivational talks so that when you feel like

giving up you have a new reason to start working out again.
Most people have trouble asking for help but it is vital to remember that it is okay to lean on others when you need to.

You can also consider joining a social networking site or an online community where other people are also trying to reduce fat so that you can share your issues and learn from their mistakes and not repeat them. Doing stuff with other people keeps you motivated and it makes it much more fun.

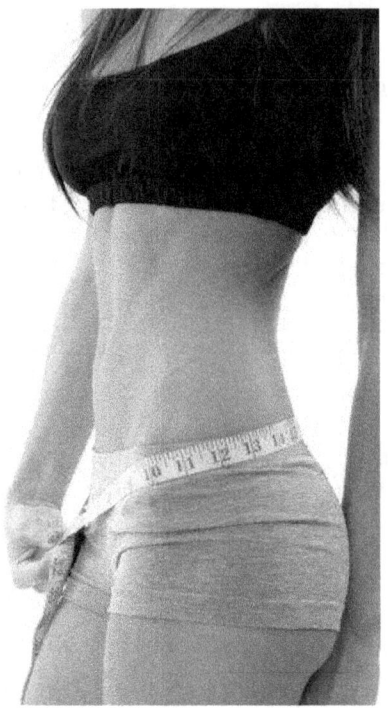

Conclusion

Fear of failure is worse than the failure itself. To achieve a healthy body, discard the factor of laziness and no-time-for-it approach from the equation of your life. Include working on both physical and mental grounds. Make sure to follow a diet chart which eliminates all sorts of junk food and fizzy drinks from your balanced diet.

The possibility of suffering from severe health problems are much higher when a person is overweight or under uncontrollable obesity.

Always give maximum attention to foods like:

- vegetables
- fruits
- bran
- leafy vegetables
- fish
- nuts
- fruit shakes
- meat along with 8 to 10 glasses of water daily.

It is very advisable to have your own healthy recipes. The main reason for poor health, fatigue and longtime sickness is the improper, imbalanced and irrational eating habits. A lot of people these days suffer from diabetes, cancer and obesity just because of poor attention they give to their eating habits and routine.

To keep the machine running you really need to keep running. It is very beneficial to exercise at least 30-40 minutes 5 days a week. Early morning exercises can help you achieve a refreshed and exhilarating day full of energy and enthusiasm. Involving in variety of exercises is very much appreciable, like swimming, jogging, trekking, horse riding, sprinting, biking or even simple walking. Always go for activities that interest you the most, because keeping your mind healthy is equally the part of your health strategy.

....

www.ingramcontent.com/pod-product-compliance
Lightning Source LLC
Chambersburg PA
CBHW070339290526
45791CB00003B/1395